Keto Cookbook for Busy People

Easy, Simple & Basic Ketogenic Diet Recipes

Haya Mays

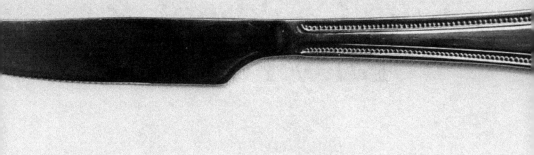

KETO DIET

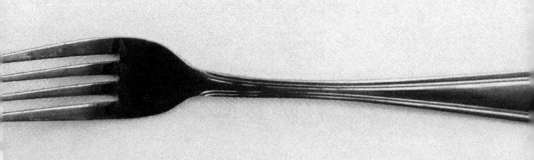

CONTENTS

TASTY BREAKFAST RECIPES 9

Microwave Bacon Mug Eggs 11

Egg & Avocado Ratatouille 12

Hard-Boiled Eggs with Tuna & Chili Mayo...........14

Lazy Eggs with Feta Cheese................................16

Breakfast Serrano Ham Frittata with Salad.........17

Bell Pepper Frittata with Cheese & Dill...............19

Asparagus & Goat Cheese Frittata 20

Sour Cream Crabmeat Frittata with Onion 22

Chorizo & Cheese Frittata 24

Italian-Style Croque Madame 26

HEALTHY SALADS & SOUPS 28

Feat Salad with Broccoli & Spinach 29

Tomato & Colby Cheese Salad 30

Iceberg Lettuce Salad with Bacon 31

Mushroom & Pepper Salad................................32

Cauliflower & Watercress Salad.........................34

Tofu & Collard Green Salad................................35

Caprese Salad Stacks with Anchovies 36

Asparagus & Green Bean Salad..........................37

Green Squash Salad...38

Summer Gazpacho with Cottage Cheese.............39

JUICY POULTRY..41

Cheesy Pinwheels with Chicken.................................42

Winter Chicken with Vegetables 44

Marinated Fried Chicken 47

Mediterranean Stuffed Chicken Breasts....................48

Zucchini & Bell Pepper Chicken Gratin 50

Juicy Chicken with Broccoli & Pine Nuts................52

Chili Chicken Kebab with Garlic Dressing...............54

Awesome Chicken Kabobs with Celery Root Chips 56

Pan-Fried Chicken with Anchovy Tapenade 58

Pancetta & Cheese Stuffed Chicken 59

Fennel & Chicken Wrapped in Bacon 60

Feta & Bacon Chicken 62

FISH & SEAFOOD 63

Catalan Shrimp with Garlic 64

Shirataki Noodles with Shrimp & Cheese 65

Zucchini Stuffed with Shrimp & Tomato................67

Coconut Fried Shrimp with Cilantro Sauce 68

Chimichurri Tiger Shrimp 70

Mustardy Crab Cakes 72

Spicy Mussels with Shirataki Pasta 73

Mussel Coconut Curry.......................................75

Pan-Seared Scallops with Sausage........................77

DESSERTS 78

Fluffy Lemon Curd Mousse with Walnuts...............79

Chocolate Mousse with Cherries 81

Grandma's Coconut Treats....................................84

Chocolate Almond Ice Cream Treats....................86

Creamy Berry Bowl with Pecans 88

Hot Chocolate with Almonds & Cinnamon 89

Winter Hot Chocolate with Peanuts 91

Minty Lemon Tart...92

Maple-Vanilla Tart..95

Lavender & Raspberry Pie....................................98

Cinnamon Pumpkin Pie 100

Fresh Berry Galette 102

Vanilla Passion Fruit Galette 105

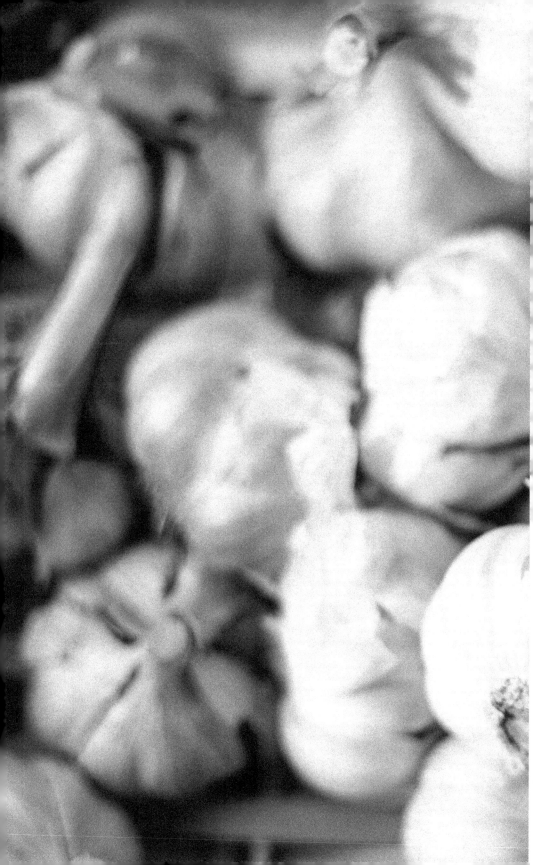

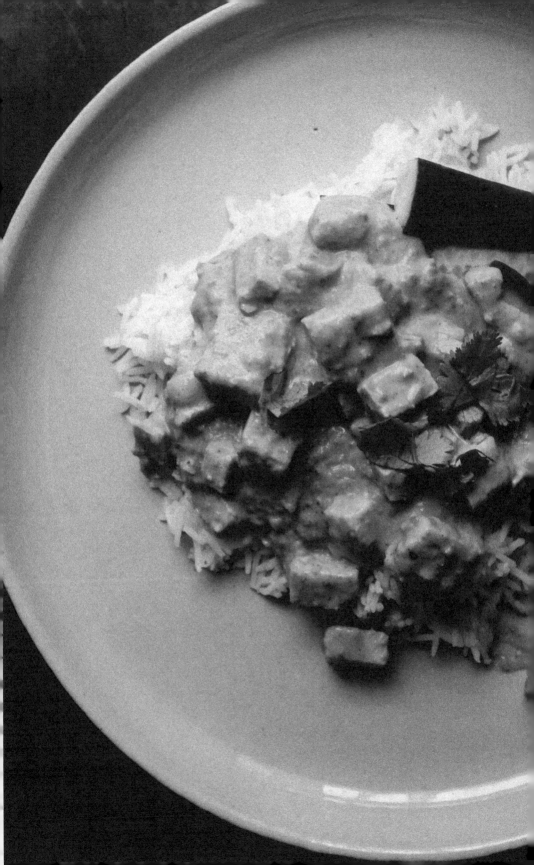

TASTY

BREAKFAST

RECIPES

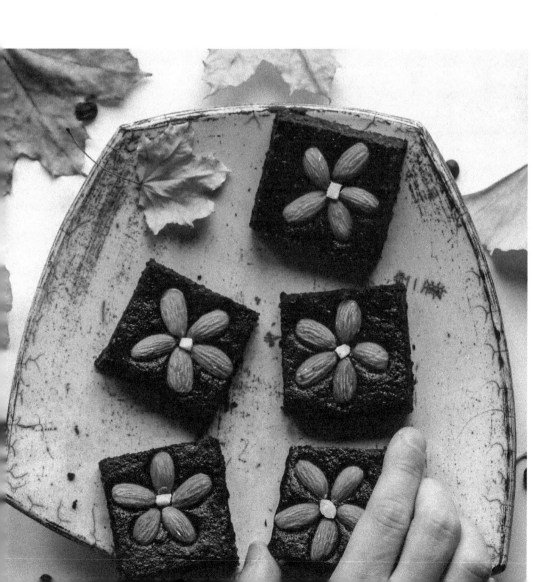

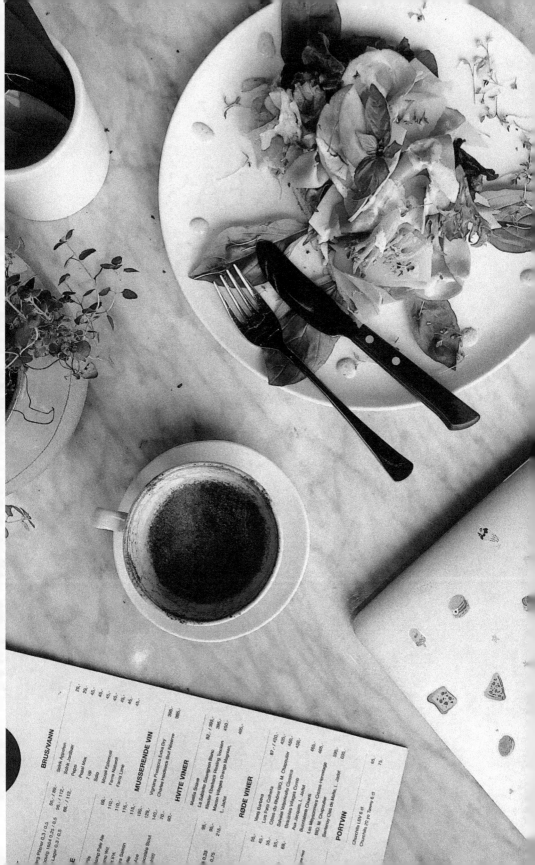

Microwave Bacon Mug Eggs

Ingredients for 2 servings
4 eggs
4 tbsp coconut milk
½ cup bacon, cubed
½ tsp oregano
Salt and black pepper, to taste
1 spring onion, sliced

Directions and Total Time: approx. 5 minutes
In a bowl, crack the eggs and beat until combined; season with salt and
black pepper.
Add coconut milk, bacon, spring onion, and oregano.
Pour the mixture into two microwave-safe cups.
Microwave for 1 minute.
Serve.

Per serving: Cal 370; Fat 17g; Net Carbs 1.9g; Protein 23g

Egg & Avocado Ratatouille

Ingredients for 2 servings
4 eggs
1 avocado, chopped
1 tbsp olive oil
1 medium red onion, sliced
1 zucchini, sliced
1 red bell pepper, sliced
1 yellow bell pepper, sliced
1 medium tomato, diced
1 cup vegetable broth
1 tbsp chopped parsley

Directions and Total Time: approx. 50 minutes
Warm olive oil in a skillet and sauté the zucchini, onion, and bell peppers
for 10 minutes.
Pour in tomato and vegetable broth.
Bring to a boil, reduce the heat, and then simmer until the sauce thickens
slightly.
Create four holes in the sauce and break an egg into each hole.
Allow the eggs to cook through and turn the heat off.
Plate the sauce, top with the avocado and parsley.
Serve.

Per serving: Cal 448; Net Carbs 5.6g; Fat 29g; Protein 18g

Hard-Boiled Eggs with Tuna & Chili Mayo

Ingredients for 4 servings
4 eggs
14 oz tuna in brine, drained
½ small head lettuce, torn
2 spring onions, chopped
¼ cup ricotta, crumbled
2 tbsp sour cream
½ tbsp mustard powder
½ cup mayonnaise
½ tbsp lemon juice
½ tbsp chili powder
2 dill pickles, sliced
Salt and black pepper, to taste

Directions and Total Time: approx. 20 minutes
Boil the eggs in salted water over medium heat for 10 minutes.
Place in an ice bath, cool and chop into small pieces.
Transfer it to a bowl and set aside.
Place in tuna, onion, mustard powder, ricotta cheese, lettuce, and sour
cream.
In a separate bowl, mix in mayonnaise, lemon juice, and chili powder.
Add in pepper and salt.
Add in the tuna mixture and stir to combine well.
Serve topped with dill pickle slices.

Per serving: Cal 311; Fat 19g; Net Carbs 1.5g;
Protein 31g

Lazy Eggs with Feta Cheese

Ingredients for 2 servings
4 eggs
¼ cup coconut milk
¼ cup feta cheese, grated
1 garlic clove, minced
¼ tsp dried dill
¼ tsp red pepper flakes

Directions and Total Time: approx. 5 minutes
Beat the eggs lightly with a fork in a bowl.
Mix in the feta, red pepper flakes, garlic, coconut milk, and salt.
Divide the mixture between greased microwave-safe mugs.
Microwave the mugs for 40 seconds.
Stir well and continue microwaving for 70 seconds.
Sprinkle with dill.

Per serving: Cal 234; Fat 16g; Net Carbs 2.7g; Protein 17g

Breakfast Serrano Ham Frittata with Salad

Ingredients for 2 servings
2 tbsp extra virgin olive oil
3 slices serrano ham, chopped
1 tomato, cut into chunks
1 cucumber, sliced
1 small red onion, sliced
1 tbsp balsamic vinegar
4 eggs
1 cup Swiss chard, chopped
Salt and black pepper to tastc
1 green onion, sliced

Directions and Total Time: approx. 22 minutes
Whisk vinegar, 1 tbsp of olive oil, salt, and pepper
to make the dressing; set
aside.
Combine tomato, red onion, and cucumber in a
salad bowl, drizzle with the
dressing and toss the veggies.
Sprinkle with serrano ham.
Crack the eggs into a bowl.
Season with salt and pepper.
Heat the remaining olive oil in the pan over
medium heat.
Sauté the onion for 3 minutes.
Add in the Swiss chard, season with salt and
pepper, and cook for 2
minutes.

Pour the egg mixture all over the Swiss chard, reduce the heat to mediumlow,
cover, and cook for 4 minutes.
Transfer the pan to the oven.
Bake to brown on top for 5 minutes at 390 F.
Serve the frittata with the salad.

Per serving: Cal 364; Fat 26g; Net Carbs 4.7g; Protein 20g

Bell Pepper Frittata with Cheese & Dill

Ingredients for 2 servings
½ green bell pepper, diced
½ cup feta cheese, crumbled
1 tomato, sliced
4 eggs
1 tbsp olive oil
2 scallions, diced
1 tsp dill, chopped
Salt and black pepper, to taste

Directions and Total Time: approx. 40 minutes
Preheat oven to 360 F.
In a bowl, whisk the eggs along with the pepper and salt, until combined.
Stir in the bell pepper, feta cheese, and scallions.
Pour the mixture into a greased casserole, top with the tomato slices and
bake for 25 minutes until the frittata is set in the middle.
Sprinkle with dill.
Serve immediately and enjoy!

Per serving: Cal 311; Fat 25g; Net Carbs 3.6g; Protein 16g

Asparagus & Goat Cheese Frittata

Ingredients for 2 servings
1 tbsp olive oil
½ onion, chopped
1 cup asparagus, chopped
4 eggs, beaten
½ habanero pepper, minced
Salt and red pepper, to taste
¾ cup goat cheese, crumbled
½ tbsp basil pesto
1 tbsp parsley, to serve

Directions and Total Time: approx. 20 minutes
Preheat oven to 370 F.
Sauté onion in warm olive oil over medium heat until caramelized.
Place in the asparagus and cook until tender, about 5 minutes.
Add in habanero pepper and eggs; season with red pepper and salt.
Cook until the eggs are set.
Scatter goat cheese over the frittata.
Transfer to the oven and cook for approximately 12 minutes, until the
frittata is set in the middle.
Slice into wedges and decorate with parsley before serving.

Per serving: Cal 345; Fat 27g; Net Carbs 5.3g; Protein 22g

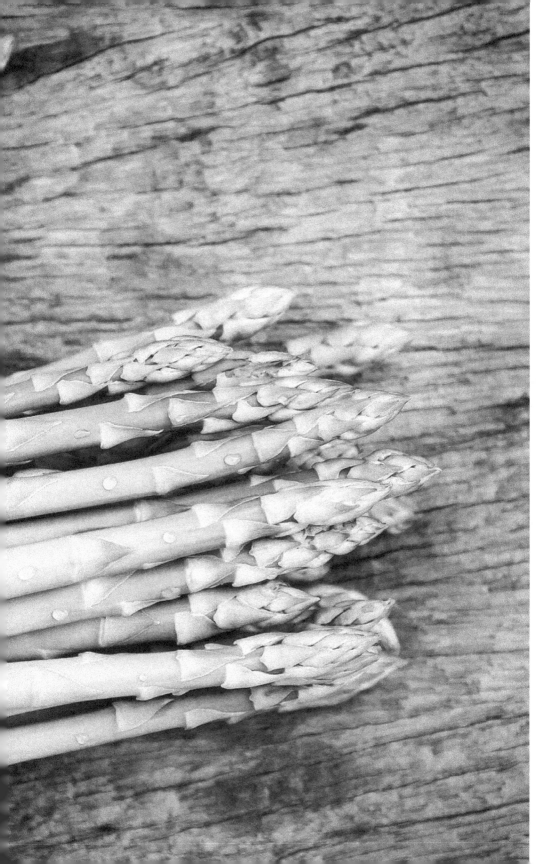

Sour Cream Crabmeat Frittata with Onion

Ingredients for 2 servings
1 tbsp olive oil
½ onion, chopped
Salt and black pepper to taste
½ tsp cilantro
3 oz crabmeat, chopped
1 tsp cajun seasoning
4 large eggs, slightly beaten
½ cup sour cream

Directions and Total Time: approx. 25 minutes
Put a large skillet over medium heat and warm the oil.
Add in onion and sauté until soft; place in crabmeat and cook for 2 more
minutes.
Season with salt and pepper.
Distribute the ingredients at the bottom of the skillet.
Whisk the eggs with sour cream.
Transfer to the skillet.
Set the skillet in the oven and bake for about 18 minutes at 350 F or until
eggs are cooked through.
Slice into wedges and serve warm.

Per serving: Cal 265; Fat 16g; Net Carbs 6.5g; Protein 23g

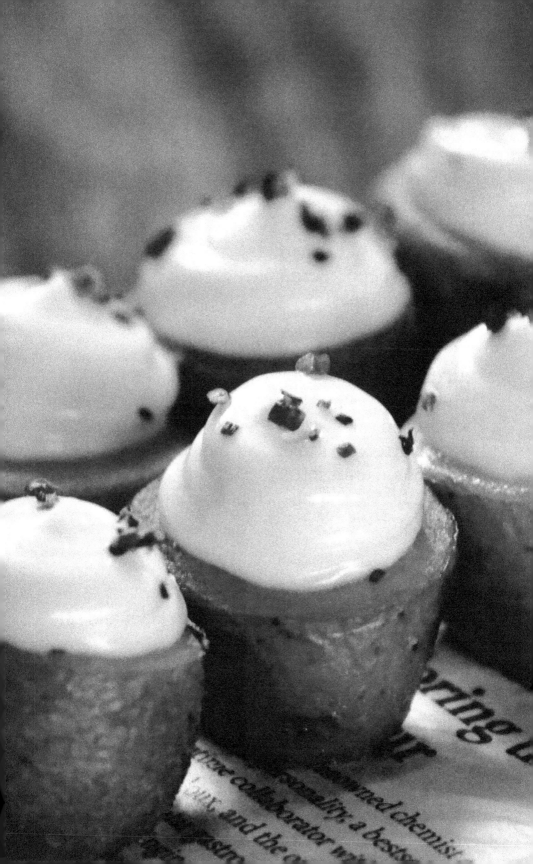

Chorizo & Cheese Frittata

Ingredients for 2 servings

4 eggs
Salt and black pepper, to taste
1 chorizo sausage, sliced
1 tbsp butter
1 green onion, chopped
½ red bell pepper, crumbled
1 tsp chipotle paste
½ cup kale
¼ cup cotija cheese, shredded

Directions and Total Time: approx. 25 minutes

Whisk the eggs in a bowl, and season with black pepper and salt.
Warm butter in a skillet over medium heat.
Sauté onion until soft.
Add in chorizo sausage, chipotle paste, and bell pepper, and cook for 5-7
minutes.
Place in kale and cook for 2 minutes.
Add in the eggs.
Spread the mixture evenly over the skillet and set to the oven.
Bake for 8 minutes at 370 F or until the top is set and golden.
Scatter crumbled cotija cheese over and bake for 3 more minutes or until
the cheese melts completely.

Slice and serve while still warm.

Per serving: Cal 288; Fat 21g; Net Carbs 5.3g; Protein 17g

Italian-Style Croque Madame

Ingredients for 4 servings

1 (7-oz) can sliced mushrooms, drained
4 tbsp melted butter
4 tbsp grated Monterey Jack
¼ cup grated Parmesan
1 cup + 2 tbsp almond milk
Salt and black pepper to taste
½ tsp nutmeg powder
½ cup basil leaves
1/3 cup toasted pine nuts
1 garlic clove, peeled
¼ cup + 1 tbsp olive oil
3 medium tomatoes, sliced
4 slices mozzarella cheese
4 large whole eggs
4 slices zero carb bread
Baby arugula for garnishing

Directions and Total Time: approx. 45 minutes

Add half of the butter and half of the milk to a saucepan over medium heat.
Whisk in the remaining milk with flour until smooth roux forms.
Season with salt, pepper, and nutmeg.
Reduce the heat and stir in Monterey Jack cheese until melted.
Set aside the bechamel sauce.

For the pesto, in a food processor, puree basil, pine nuts, Parmesan
cheese, garlic, and ¼ cup olive oil.
Refrigerate the resulting pesto.
Preheat grill to medium-high.
Brush both sides of each bread slice with remaining butter.
Toast each on both sides.
Remove onto a plate and spread béchamel sauce on one side of each
bread, then pesto, and top with tomatoes and mozzarella cheese.
One after the other, return each sandwich to the grill and cook until the
cheese melts.
Heat the remaining olive oil in a skillet and crack in eggs.
Cook until the whites set but the yolks still soft and runny.
Place the eggs on the sandwiches.
Garnish with arugula.

Per serving: Cal 628; Net Carbs 3.8g; Fat 58g; Protein 25g

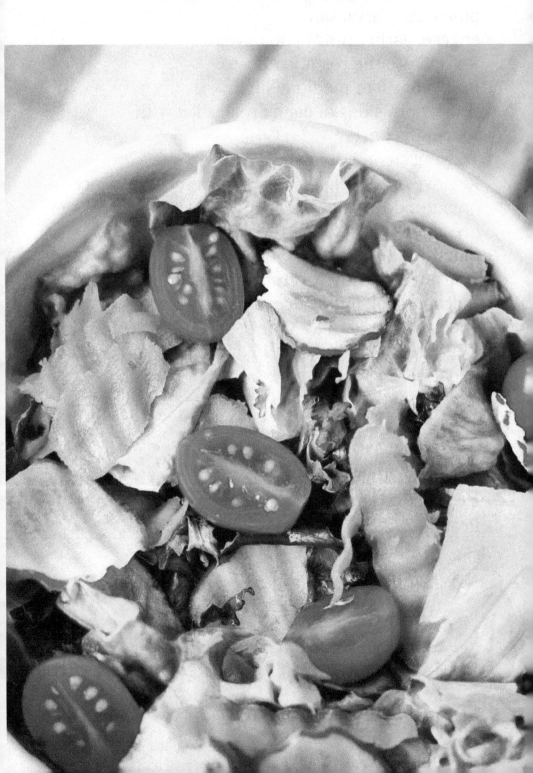

Feat Salad with Broccoli & Spinach

Ingredients for 4 servings
2 cups broccoli slaw
2 cups chopped spinach
2 tbsp poppy seeds
1/3 cup sunflower seeds
1/3 cup blueberries
2/3 cup chopped feta cheese
1/3 cup chopped walnuts
2 tbsp olive oil
1 tbsp white wine vinegar
Salt and black pepper to taste

Directions and Total Time: approx. 15 minutes
In a bowl, whisk olive oil, vinegar, poppy seeds, salt, and pepper; set aside.
In a salad bowl, combine the broccoli slaw, spinach, walnuts, sunflower
seeds, blueberries, and feta cheese.
Drizzle the dressing on top, toss, and serve.

Per serving: Cal 401; Net Carbs 4.9g; Fat 4g; Protein 9g

Tomato & Colby Cheese Salad

Ingredients for 2 servings
½ cucumber, sliced
2 tomatoes, sliced
½ yellow bell pepper, sliced
½ red onion, sliced thinly
½ cup colby cheese, cubed
10 green olives, pitted
½ tbsp red wine vinegar
4 tbsp olive oil
½ tsp dried oregano
Salt and black pepper to serve

Directions and Total Time: approx. 10 minutes
Place the bell pepper, tomatoes, cucumber, red onion, and colby cheese in
a bowl.
Drizzle red wine vinegar and olive oil all over and season with salt, pepper,
and oregano; toss to coat.
Top with olives and serve.

Per serving: Cal 578; Net Carbs 13g; Fat 51g; Protein 15g

Iceberg Lettuce Salad with Bacon

Ingredients for 4 servings
1 ½ cups gorgonzola cheese, crumbled
1 head lettuce, separated into leaves
4 oz bacon
1 tbsp white wine vinegar
3 tbsp extra virgin olive oil
Salt and black pepper to taste
2 tbsp pumpkin seeds

Directions and Total Time: approx. 15 minutes
Chop the bacon into small pieces and fry in a skillet over medium heat for 6
minutes, until browned and crispy.
In a small bowl, whisk the white wine vinegar, olive oil, salt, and black
pepper until dressing is well combined.
To assemble the salad, arrange the lettuce on a serving platter, top with the
bacon and gorgonzola cheese.
Drizzle the dressing over the salad, lightly toss, and top with pumpkin
seeds to serve.

Per serving: Cal 339; Fat 32g; Net Carbs 2.9g; Protein 16g

Mushroom & Pepper Salad

Ingredients for 4 servings

1 cup mixed mushrooms, chopped
2 tbsp sesame oil
2 yellow bell peppers, sliced
1 garlic clove, minced
2 tbsp tamarind sauce
½ tsp hot sauce
1 tsp sugar-free maple syrup
½ tsp ginger paste
Chopped toasted pecans
Sesame seeds to garnish
Salt and black pepper to taste

Directions and Total Time: approx. 20 minutes

Warm half of the sesame oil in a skillet over medium heat and sauté bell
peppers and mushrooms for 8-10 minutes.
Season with salt and pepper.
In a bowl, mix garlic, tamarind sauce, hot sauce, maple syrup, and ginger
paste.
Stir the mix into the vegetables and stir-fry for 2-3 minutes.
Drizzle the salad with the remaining sesame oil and garnish with pecans
and sesame seeds.
Serve.

Per serving: Cal 291; Net Carbs 5.2g; Fat 27g; Protein 4.2g

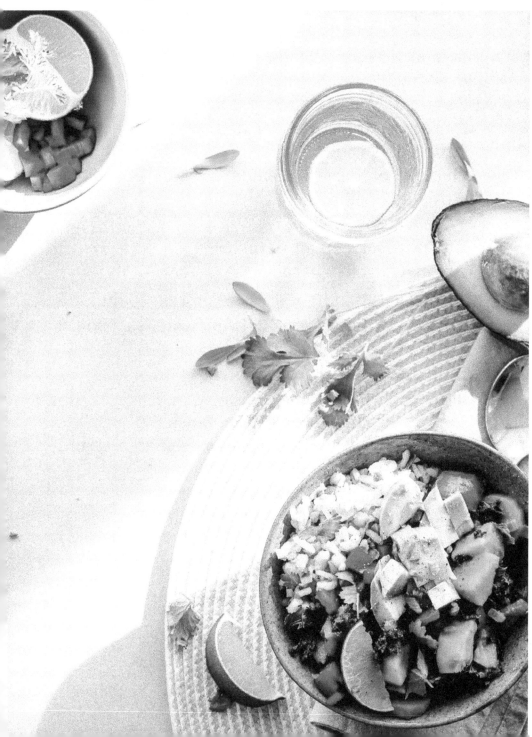

Cauliflower & Watercress Salad

Ingredients for 4 servings

2 tbsp sesame oil
1 lemon, zested and juiced
10 oz cauliflower florets
12 green olives, chopped
8 sun-dried tomatoes, drained
3 tbsp chopped scallions
A handful of toasted peanuts
3 tbsp chopped parsley
½ cup watercress
Salt and black pepper to taste
Lemon wedges to garnish

Directions and Total Time: approx. 20 minutes

Ina pot over medium heat, bring water to a boil.
Insert a steamer basket and pour in the cauliflower.
Soften for 8 minutes.
Transfer cauliflower to a salad bowl.
Add in olives, tomatoes, scallions, lemon zest and juice, sesame oil,
peanuts, parsley, and watercress.
Season with salt and pepper and mix using a spoon.
Serve with lemon wedges.

Per serving: Cal 198; Net Carbs 6.4g; Fat 15g; Protein 6.6g

Tofu & Collard Green Salad

Ingredients for 2 servings
1 cup collard greens, rinsed
4 oz tofu cheese
2 tbsp coconut oil
¾ cup coconut cream
2 tbsp mayonnaise
1 tsp mustard powder
1 garlic clove, minced
1 tbsp butter

Directions and Total Time: approx. 10 minutes
In a bowl, whisk whipping cream, mayonnaise, mustard powder, coconut
oil, garlic, salt, and pepper until well mixed; set aside.
Melt butter in a skillet over medium heat and sauté collard greens until
wilted and brownish.
Transfer to a salad bowl and pour the creamy dressing over.
Mix the salad well and crumble the tofu over.

Per serving: Cal 502; Net Carbs 5g; Fat 39g; Protein 11g

Caprese Salad Stacks with Anchovies

Ingredients for 4 servings
4 anchovy fillets in oil
12 fresh mozzarella slices
4 red tomato slices
4 yellow tomato slices
1 cup basil pesto

Directions and Total Time: approx. 10 minutes
Take a serving platter and alternately stack a
tomato slice, a mozzarella
slice, an yellow tomato slice, another mozzarella
slice, a red tomato slice,
and then a mozzarella slice on it.
Repeat making 3 more stacks in the same way.
Spoon pesto all over.
Arrange anchovies on top and serve.

Per serving: Cal 182; Net Carbs 3.5g; Fat 6g; Protein 17g

Asparagus & Green Bean Salad

Ingredients for 4 servings
2 tbsp butter
2 tbsp olive oil
1 cup green beans, trimmed
1 cup asparagus, halved
7 oz Swiss cheese, cubed
4 tbsp chopped almonds
½ lemon, juiced
Salt and black pepper to taste

Directions and Total Time: approx. 25 minutes
Melt butter in a skillet over medium heat and pour in green beans and asparagus.
Season with salt and pepper and cook until softened, about 5-8 minutes.
Remove to a serving plate.
Drizzle with lemon juice and scatter almonds and Swiss cheese on top.
Serve warm.

Per serving: Cal 241; Net Carbs 3.9g; Fat 15g; Protein 13g

Green Squash Salad

Ingredients for 4 servings
2 tbsp butter
2 lb green squash, cubed
1 fennel bulb, sliced
2 oz chopped green onions
1 cup mayonnaise
2 tbsp chives, finely chopped
2 tbsp chopped dill
A pinch of mustard powder

Directions and Total Time: approx. 20 minutes
Place a pan over medium heat and melt butter.
Fry squash until slightly softened, about 7
minutes; let cool.
In a bowl, mix squash, fennel, green onions,
mayonnaise, chives, and
mustard powder.
Garnish with dill.

Per serving: Cal 321; Net Carbs 3g; Fat 31g;
Protein 4g

Summer Gazpacho with Cottage Cheese

Ingredients for 4 servings

1 green pepper, roasted
1 red pepper, roasted
1 avocado, flesh scoped out
1 garlic clove
1 spring onion, chopped
1 cucumber, chopped
½ cup olive oil
1 tbsp lemon juice
2 tomatoes, chopped
4 oz cottage cheese, crumbled
1 small red onion, chopped
1 tbsp apple cider vinegar
Salt to taste

Directions and Total Time: approx. 15 min + cooling time

In a blender, put the peppers, tomatoes, avocados, red onion, garlic, lemon
juice, olive oil, vinegar, half of the cucumber, a cup of water, and cottage
cheese.
Blitz until your desired consistency is reached; adjust the seasoning.
Transfer the mixture to a pot.
Cover and chill in the fridge for at least 2 hours.
Serve the soup topped with the remaining cucumber, spring onion, and an

extra drizzle of olive oil.

Per serving: Cal 373; Fat 34g; Net Carbs 7.1g; Protein 5.8g

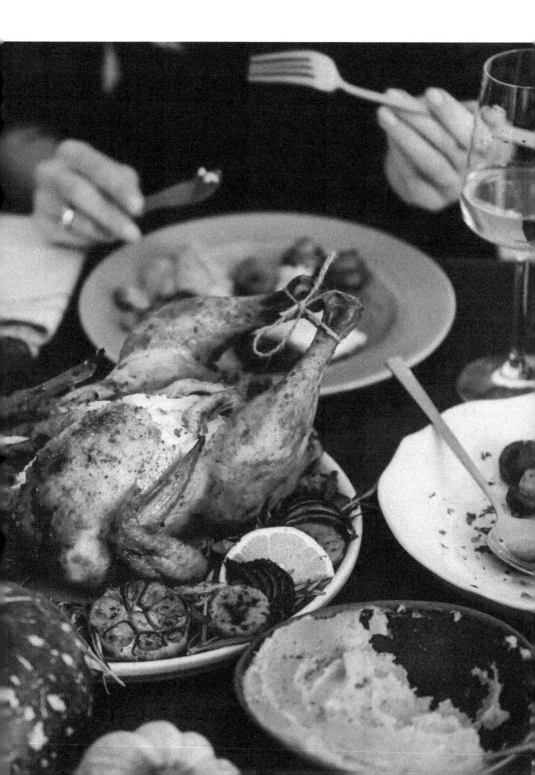

Cheesy Pinwheels with Chicken

Ingredients for 2 servings

2 tbsp ghee
1 garlic, minced
1/3 lb chicken breasts, cubed
1 tsp creole seasoning
1/3 red onion, chopped
1 tomato, chopped
½ cup chicken stock
¼ cup whipping cream
½ cup mozzarella, grated
¼ cup fresh cilantro, chopped
Salt and black pepper, to taste
4 oz cream cheese
5 eggs
A pinch of garlic powder

Directions and Total Time: approx. 30 minutes

Season the chicken with creole seasoning.

Heat a pan over medium heat and warm 1 tbsp ghee.

Add chicken and cook each side for 2 minutes; remove to a plate.

Melt the rest of the ghee and stir in garlic and tomato; cook for 4 minutes.

Return the chicken to the pan and pour in stock; cook for 15 minutes.

Place in whipping cream, red onion, salt, mozzarella cheese, and black pepper; cook for 2 minutes.

In a blender, combine cream cheese with garlic powder, salt, eggs, and

black pepper, and pulse well.

Place the mixture into a lined baking sheet, and then bake for 10 minutes in

the oven at 320 F.

Allow the cheese sheet to cool down, place on a cutting board, roll, and

slice into medium slices.

Arrange the slices on a serving plate and top with chicken mixture.

Sprinkle with cilantro to serve.

Per serving: Cal 463; Fat 36g; Net Carbs 6.3g; Protein 35g

Winter Chicken with Vegetables

Ingredients for 2 servings

2 tbsp olive oil
2 cups whipping cream
1 lb chicken breasts, chopped
1 onion, chopped
1 carrot, chopped
2 cups chicken stock
Salt and black pepper, to taste
1 bay leaf
1 turnip, chopped
1 parsnip, chopped
1 cup green beans, chopped
2 tsp fresh thyme, chopped

Directions and Total Time: approx. 35 minutes

Heat a pan over medium heat and warm the olive oil.
Sauté the onion for 3 minutes, pour in the stock, carrot, turnip, parsnip,
chicken, and bay leaf.
Bring to a boil, and simmer for 20 minutes.
Add in the asparagus and cook for 7 minutes.
Discard the bay leaf, stir in the whipping cream, adjust the taste and scatter
with thyme to serve.

Per serving: Cal 483; Fat 32g; Net Carbs 6.9g; Protein 33g

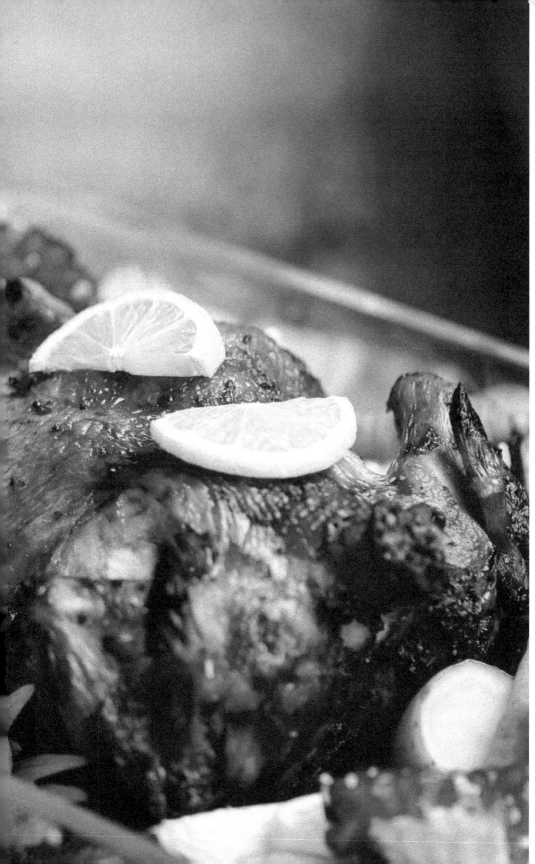

Marinated Fried Chicken

Ingredients for 2 servings
3 tbsp olive oil
2 chicken breasts, cut into strips
½ cup pork rinds, crushed
8 oz jarred pickle juice
1 egg

Directions and Total Time: approx. 20 minutes
Cover the chicken with pickle juice, in a bowl,
and refrigerate for 12 hours
while covered.
Whisk the egg in one bowl, and place the pork
rinds in a separate one.
Dip the chicken pieces in the egg, then in pork
rinds.
Ensure they are well coated.
Set a pan over medium heat and warm oil, fry the
chicken for 3 minutes on
each side, remove to paper towels, drain the
excess grease and serve.

Per serving: Cal 393; Fat 16g; Net Carbs 3.1g; Protein 21g

Mediterranean Stuffed Chicken Breasts

Ingredients for 2 servings
1 tbsp olive oil
1 cup spinach, chopped
2 chicken breasts
Salt and black pepper, to taste
½ cup cream cheese, softened
½ cup goat cheese, crumbled
1 garlic clove, minced
½ cup white wine
1 tbsp rosemary, chopped

Directions and Total Time: approx. 30 minutes
Wilt the spinach in a saucepan with a half cup of water.
Drain and mix in a bowl with the goat cheese, cream cheese, salt, garlic,
black pepper and spinach.
Cut a pocket in each chicken breast and stuff with the spinach mixture.
Preheat oven to 400 F and grease a baking tray with cooking spray.
Set a pan over medium heat and warm oil, add the stuffed chicken, and
cook each side for 5 minutes.
Then, put in the baking tray and drizzle with white wine and 2 tablespoons
of water.

Bake in the oven for 20 minutes until no more pink.

When ready, slice in half and serve sprinkled with rosemary.

Per serving: Cal 305; Fat 12g; Net Carbs 4g; Protein 23g

Zucchini & Bell Pepper Chicken Gratin

Ingredients for 2 servings
1 red bell pepper, sliced
1 zucchini, chopped
Salt and black pepper, to taste
1 tsp garlic powder
1 tbsp olive oil
2 chicken breasts, sliced
1 tomato, chopped
½ tsp dried oregano
½ tsp dried basil
½ cup mozzarella cheese, shredded

Directions and Total Time: approx. 45 minutes
Coat the chicken with salt, black pepper and garlic powder.
Warm olive oil in a skillet over medium heat and add in the chicken slices.
Cook until golden and remove to a baking dish.
To the same pan, add the zucchini, tomato, bell pepper, basil, oregano, and
salt, cook for 2 minutes, and spread over the chicken.
Bake in the oven at 360 F for 20 minutes.
Sprinkle the mozzarella over the chicken, return to the oven, and bake for 5
minutes until the cheese is melted and bubbling.

Per serving: Cal 467; Fat 23.5g; Net Carbs 6.2g; Protein 45.7g

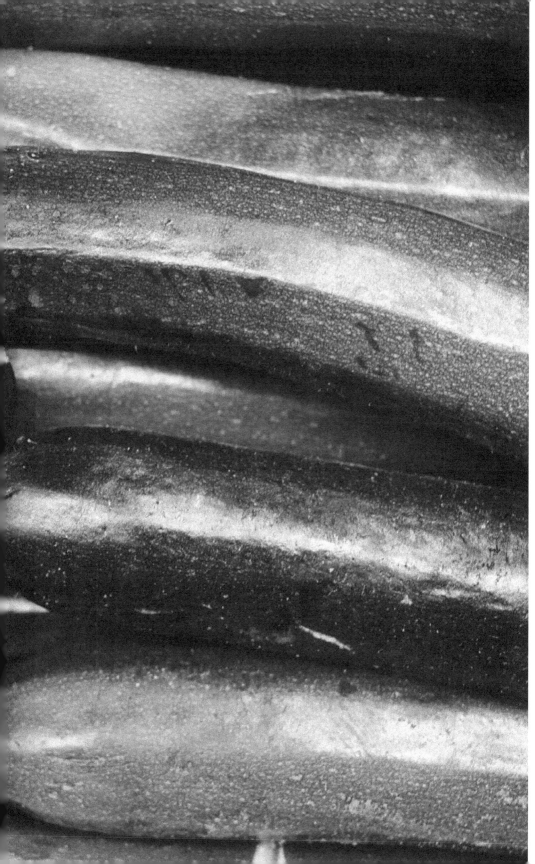

Juicy Chicken with Broccoli & Pine Nuts

Ingredients for 4 servings

2 tbsp olive oil
2 chicken breasts, cut into strips
2 tbsp Worcestershire sauce
2 tsp balsamic vinegar
2 tsp xanthan gum
1 lemon, juiced
1 cup pine nuts
2 cups broccoli florets
1 onion, thinly sliced
Salt and black pepper to taste
1 tbsp cilantro, chopped

Directions and Total Time: approx. 30 minutes

In a dry pan over medium heat, toast the pine
nuts for 2 minutes until
golden-brown; set aside.
To the pan, add olive oil and sauté the onion for 4
minutes until soft and
browned; remove to the nuts.
In a bowl, mix the Worcestershire sauce,
balsamic vinegar, lemon juice,
and xanthan gum; set aside.
Add the chicken to the pan and cook for 4
minutes.
Add in the broccoli, salt, and black pepper.
Stir-fry and pour in the lemon mixture in.

Cook the sauce for 4 minutes and pour in the pine nuts and onion.

Stir once more and cook for 1 minute.

Serve the chicken stir-fry with cilantro.

Per serving: Cal 286; Fat 10.1g; Net Carbs 3.4g; Protein 17.3g

Chili Chicken Kebab with Garlic Dressing

Ingredients for 4 servings

Skewers
2 tbsp olive oil
3 tbsp soy sauce, sugar-free
1 tbsp ginger paste
2 tbsp swerve brown sugar
Chili pepper to taste
2 chicken breasts, cut into cubes
Dressing
½ cup tahini
1 tbsp parsley, chopped
1 garlic clove, minced
Salt and black pepper to taste
¼ cup warm water

Directions and Total Time: approx. 17 min + cooling time

To make the marinade, in a small bowl, whisk the soy sauce, ginger paste,
brown sugar, chili pepper, and olive oil.
Put the chicken in a zipper bag, pour the marinade over, seal and shake for
an even coat.
Marinate in the fridge for 2 hours.
Preheat a grill to high heat.
Thread the chicken on skewers and cook for 10 minutes in total with three
to four turnings to be golden brown.

Transfer to a plate.

Mix the tahini, garlic, salt, parsley, and warm water in a bowl.

Serve the chicken skewers topped with the tahini dressing.

Per serving: Cal 410; Fat 32g; Net Carbs 4.8g; Protein 23.5g

Awesome Chicken Kabobs with Celery Root Chips

Ingredients for 2 servings
4 tbsp olive oil
2 chicken breasts
Salt and black pepper to taste
1 tsp dried oregano
1 tsp chili powder
¼ cup chicken broth
1 lb celery root, sliced

Directions and Total Time: approx. 60 minutes
Preheat oven to 400 F and grease a baking sheet with cooking spray.
In a large bowl, mix half of the olive oil, oregano, chili powder, salt, black
pepper, and the chicken; set in the fridge for 10 minutes.
Arrange the celery slices on the baking tray in an even layer, drizzle with
the remaining olive oil and sprinkle with salt and black pepper.
Bake for 10 minutes.
Take the chicken from the refrigerator and thread onto skewers.
Place over the celery, pour in the chicken broth, then set in the oven for 30
minutes.

Per serving: Cal 365; Fat 23g; Net Carbs 4.6g; Protein 35g

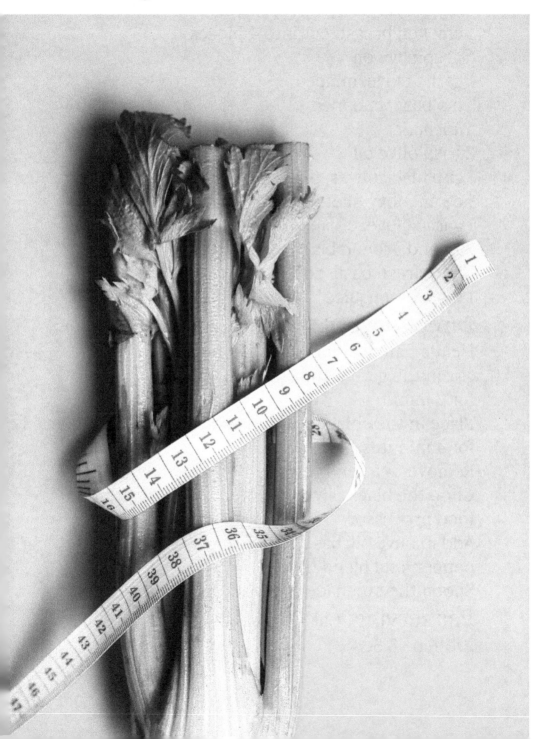

Pan-Fried Chicken with Anchovy Tapenade

Ingredients for 2 servings
1 chicken breast, cut into 4 pieces
2 tbsp olive oil
1 garlic clove, minced
1 tsp basil, chopped
Tapenade
2 tbsp olive oil
1 cup black olives, pitted
1 oz anchovy fillets, rinsed
1 garlic clove, crushed
Salt and ground black pepper, to taste
¼ cup fresh basil, chopped
1 tbsp lemon juice

Directions and Total Time: approx. 30 minutes
Heat a pan over medium heat and add olive oil, stir in the garlic, and cook
for 2 minutes.
Place in the chicken pieces and cook each side
for 4 minutes.
Remove to a serving plate.
Chop the black olives and anchovy and put in a food processor.
Add in olive oil, basil, lemon juice, salt, and black pepper, and blend well.
Spoon the tapenade over the chicken to serve.

Per serving: Cal 522; Fat 37.3g; Net Carbs 5.3g; Protein 43.5g

Pancetta & Cheese Stuffed Chicken

Ingredients for 2 servings

4 slices pancetta
2 tbsp olive oil
2 chicken breasts
1 garlic clove, minced
1 shallot, finely chopped
2 tbsp dried oregano
4 oz mascarpone cheese
1 lemon, zested
Salt and black pepper to taste

Directions and Total Time: approx. 40 minutes

Heat the oil in a small skillet and sauté the garlic and shallots for 3 minutes.
Stir in salt, black pepper, and lemon zest.
Transfer to a bowl and let it cool.
Stir in the mascarpone cheese and oregano.
Score a pocket in each chicken's breast, fill the holes with the cheese
mixture and cover with the cut-out chicken.
Wrap each breast with two pancetta slices and secure the ends with a
toothpick.
Lay the chicken on a greased baking sheet and cook in the oven for 20
minutes at 380 F.

Per serving: Cal 643; Fat 44.5g; Net Carbs 6.2g; Protein 52.8g

Fennel & Chicken Wrapped in Bacon

Ingredients for 4 servings
2 tbsp olive oil
2 chicken breasts
Salt and black pepper to taste
½ lb bacon, sliced
½ lb fennel bulb, sliced
2 tbsp lemon juice
2 tbsp cheddar cheese, shredded
1 tbsp rosemary, chopped

Directions and Total Time: approx. 48 minutes
Preheat your grill on high heat.
Brush the fennel slices with olive oil and season with salt.
Grill for 4-6 minutes, frequently turning until slightly golden.
Remove to a plate and drizzle with lemon juice.
Pour over cheddar cheese so that it melts a little on contact with the hot
fennel and forms a cheesy dressing.
Preheat oven to 390 F.
Season chicken breasts with salt and black pepper, and wrap 2 bacon
slices around each chicken breast.
Arrange on a baking sheet that is lined with parchment paper, drizzle with
oil and bake for 25-30 minutes until bacon is brown and crispy.

Serve with grilled fennel sprinkled with rosemary.
Per serving: Cal 487; Fat 39.5g; Net Carbs 5.2g; Protein 27.3g

Feta & Bacon Chicken

Ingredients for 4 servings
4 oz bacon, chopped
1 lb chicken breasts
3 green onions, chopped
2 tbsp coconut oil
4 oz feta cheese, crumbled
1 tbsp parsley

Directions and Total Time: approx. 30 minutes
Place a pan over medium heat and coat with cooking spray.
Add in the bacon and cook until crispy.
Remove to paper towels, drain the grease and crumble.
To the same pan, add in the oil and cook the chicken breasts for 4-5
minutes, then flip to the other side; cook for an additional 4-5 minutes.
Add the chicken breasts to a baking dish.
Place the green onions, set in the oven, turn on the broiler, and cook for 5
minutes at high temperature.
Remove to serving plates and serve topped with bacon, feta cheese, and
parsley.

Per serving: Cal 459; Fat 35g; Net Carbs 3.1g; Protein 32g

FISH & SEAFOOD

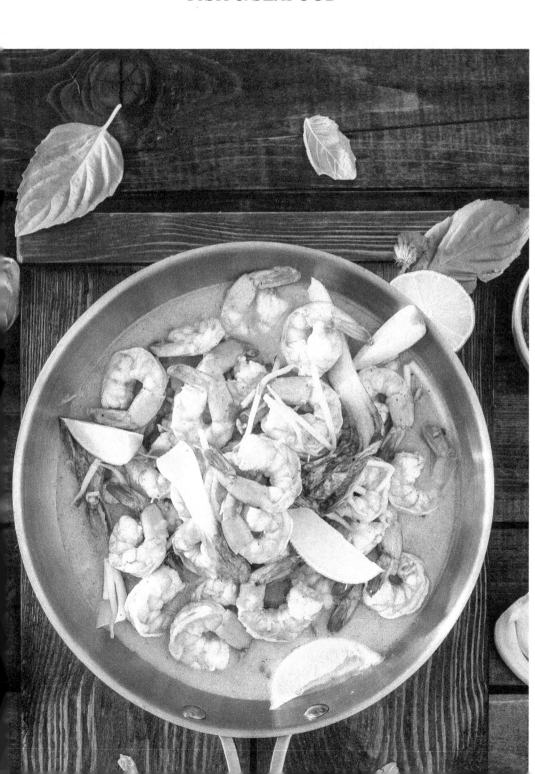

Catalan Shrimp with Garlic

Ingredients for 4 servings
¼ cup olive oil, divided
1 lb shrimp, peeled and deveined
Salt to taste
¼ tsp cayenne pepper
3 garlic cloves, sliced
2 tbsp chopped parsley

Directions and Total Time: approx. 22 minutes
Warm olive oil in a large skillet over medium heat.
Reduce the heat and add the garlic; cook for 6-8 minutes, but make sure it
doesn't brown or burn.
Add the shrimp, season with salt and cayenne pepper, stir for one minute
and turn off the heat.
Let the shrimp finish cooking with the heat of the hot oil for about 8-10
minutes.
Serve garnished with parsley.

Per serving: Cal 441; Fat 29g; Net Carbs 1.2g; Protein 43g

Shirataki Noodles with Shrimp & Cheese

Ingredients for 4 servings
1 tbsp olive oil
1 lb shrimp, deveined
8 oz angel hair shirataki noodles
2 tbsp unsalted butter
6 garlic cloves, minced
½ cup dry white wine
1 ½ cups heavy cream
½ cup grated Asiago cheese
2 tbsp chopped fresh parsley

Directions and Total Time: approx. 25 minutes
Warm olive oil in a skillet over medium heat and cook the shrimp on both
sides, 2 minutes; set aside.
Melt butter in the skillet and sauté garlic.
Stir in wine and cook until reduced by half, scraping the bottom of the pan
to deglaze.
Stir in heavy cream.
Let simmer for 1 minute and stir in Asiago cheese to melt.
Return the shrimp to the sauce and sprinkle the parsley on top.
Bring 2 cups of water to a boil.
Strain shirataki pasta and rinse under hot running water.

Allow proper draining and pour the shirataki pasta into the boiling water.

Cook for 3 minutes and strain again.

Place a dry skillet and stir-fry the pasta until dry, 1-2 minutes.

Top with the shrimp sauce and serve.

Per serving: Cal 489; Net Carbs 6g; Fats 27g; Protein 29g

Zucchini Stuffed with Shrimp & Tomato

Ingredients for 2 servings

1 lb zucchinis, tops removed and reserved
1 lb small shrimp, peeled, deveined
¼ onion, chopped
1 tsp olive oil
1 small tomato, chopped
Salt and black pepper to taste
1 tbsp basil leaves, chopped

Directions and Total Time: approx. 35 minutes

Scoop out the seeds of the zucchinis with a
spoon and set aside.
Warm olive oil in a skillet and sauté the onion and
tomato for 3 minutes.
Add the shrimp, zucchini flesh, basil leaves, salt,
and pepper and cook for
another 5 minutes.
Fill the zucchini shells with the mixture.
Cover with the zucchini tops and place them on a
greased baking sheet to
cook for 15 to 20 minutes at 390 F.
The shrimp should no longer be pink by this time.
Remove the zucchinis and serve with tomato and
mozzarella salad.

Per serving: Cal 252; Fat 6g; Net Carbs 8.9g; Protein 37.6g

Coconut Fried Shrimp with Cilantro Sauce

Ingredients for 2 servings
2 tsp coconut flour
2 tbsp grated Pecorino cheese
1 egg, beaten in a bowl
¼ tsp curry powder
½ lb shrimp, shelled
3 tbsp coconut oil
Salt to taste
Sauce
2 tbsp ghee
2 tbsp cilantro leaves, chopped
½ onion, diced
½ cup coconut cream
½ oz Paneer cheese, grated

Directions and Total Time: approx. 15 minutes
Combine coconut flour, Pecorino cheese, curry powder, and salt in a bowl.
Melt the coconut oil in a skillet over medium heat.
Dip the shrimp in the egg first, and then coat with the dry mixture.
Fry until golden and crispy, about 5 minutes.
In another skillet, melt the ghee.
Add onion and cook for 3 minutes.
Add curry and cilantro and cook for 30 seconds.
Stir in coconut cream and Paneer cheese and cook until thickened.

Add the shrimp and coat well.
Serve warm.

Per serving: Cal 741; Fat 64g; Net Carbs 4.3g; Protein 34g

Chimichurri Tiger Shrimp

Ingredients for 4 servings

1 lb tiger shrimp, peeled and deveined
2 tbsp olive oil
1 garlic clove, minced
Juice of 1 lime
Salt and black pepper to taste
Chimichurri
Salt and black pepper to taste
¼ cup extra-virgin olive oil
2 garlic cloves, minced
1 lime, juiced
¼ cup red wine vinegar
2 cups parsley, minced
¼ tsp red pepper flakes

Directions and Total Time: approx. 55 minutes

Combine the shrimp, olive oil, garlic, and lime juice, in a bowl, and let
marinate in the fridge for 30 minutes.
To make the chimichurri dressing, blitz the chimichurri ingredients in a
blender until smooth; set aside.
Preheat your grill to medium.
Add shrimp and cook for about 2 minutes per side.
Serve shrimp drizzled with the chimichurri dressing.

Per serving: Cal 523; Fat 30g; Net Carbs 7.2g; Protein 49g

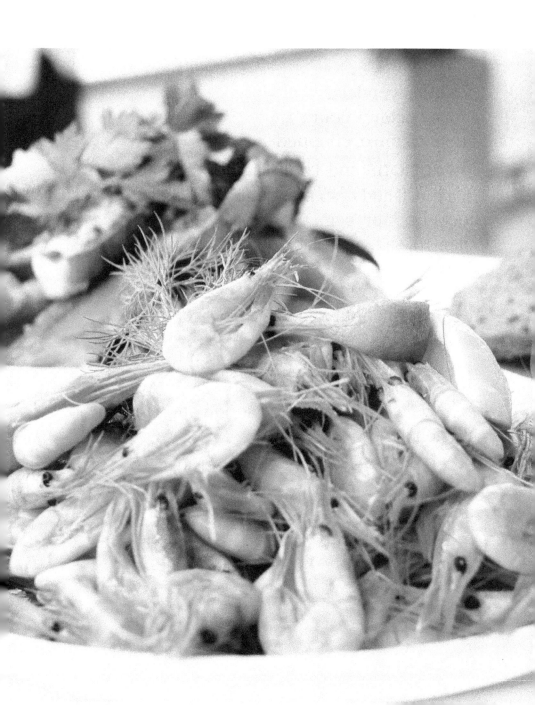

Mustardy Crab Cakes

Ingredients for 4 servings
1 tbsp coconut oil
1 lb lump crab meat
1 tsp Dijon mustard
1 egg
¼ cup mayonnaise
1 tbsp coconut flour
1 tbsp cilantro, chopped

Directions and Total Time: approx. 15 minutes
In a bowl, add crab meat, mustard, mayonnaise, coconut flour, egg,
cilantro, salt, and black pepper; mix well to combine.
Make patties out of the mixture.
Melt the coconut oil in a skillet over medium heat.
Add the crab patties and cook for about 2-3 minutes per side.
Remove with a perforated spoon and drain on kitchen paper.

Per serving: Cal 315; Fat 25g; Net Carbs 1.6g; Protein 13g

Spicy Mussels with Shirataki Pasta

Ingredients for 4 servings
4 tbsp olive oil
8 oz angel hair shirataki
1 lb mussels
1 cup white wine
6 garlic cloves, minced
3 shallots, finely chopped
2 tsp red chili flakes
½ cup fish stock
1 ½ cups heavy cream
2 tbsp chopped fresh parsley
Salt and black pepper to taste

Directions and Total Time: approx. 25 minutes
Pour 2 cups of water into a pot and bring it to a boil.
Strain the shirataki pasta and rinse well under hot running water.
Drain and transfer to the boiling water.
Cook for 3 minutes and strain again.
Place a large dry skillet and stir-fry the shirataki pasta until visibly dry, 1-2
minutes; set aside.
Pour mussels and white wine into a pot over medium heat, cover, and cook
for 3-4 minutes.
Strain mussels and reserve the cooking liquid.

Let cool, discard any closed mussels, and remove the meat out of ¾ of the
mussel shells.
Set aside the remaining mussels in the shells.
Heat olive oil in a skillet and sauté shallots, garlic, and chili flakes for 3
minutes.
Mix in reduced wine and fish stock.
Allow boiling and whisk in the heavy cream.
Season with salt, and pepper.
Pour in shirataki pasta, mussels, and toss to combine.
Top with parsley.

Per serving: Cal 469; Net Carbs 6g; Fats 34g; Protein 21g

Mussel Coconut Curry

Ingredients for 4 servings
2 tbsp cup coconut oil
2 green onions, chopped
1 lb mussels, de-bearded
1 shallot, chopped
1 garlic clove, minced
½ cup coconut milk
½ cup white wine
1 tsp red curry powder
2 tbsp parsley, chopped

Directions and Total Time: approx. 25 minutes
Cook the shallots and garlic in the wine over low heat.
Stir in the coconut milk and red curry powder and cook for 3 minutes.
Add the mussels and steam for 7 minutes or until their shells are opened.
Then, use a slotted spoon to remove to a bowl leaving the sauce in the
pan.
Discard any closed mussels at this point.
Stir the coconut oil into the sauce, turn the heat off, and stir in the parsley
and green onions.
Serve the sauce immediately with a butternut squash mash.

Per serving: Cal 356; Fat 21g; Net Carbs 0.3g; Protein 21g

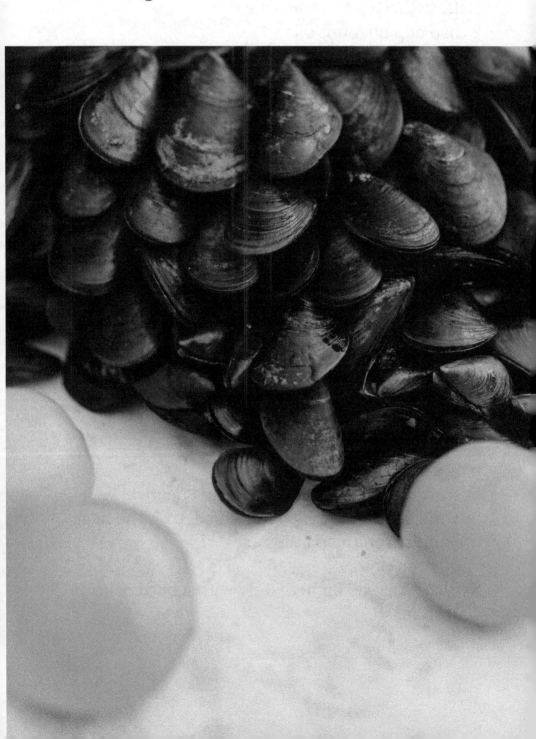

Pan-Seared Scallops with Sausage

Ingredients for 4 servings
2 tbsp butter
12 fresh scallops, rinsed
8 oz sausage, chopped
1 red bell pepper, sliced
1 red onion, finely chopped
1 cup Grana Padano, grated
Salt and black pepper to taste

Directions and Total Time: approx. 15 minutes
Melt half of the butter in a skillet over medium heat, and cook the onion and
bell pepper for 5 minutes until tender.
Add the sausage and stir-fry for another 5 minutes.
Remove and set aside.
Pat dry scallops with paper towels, and season with salt and pepper.
Add the remaining butter to the skillet and sear scallops for 2 minutes on
each side to have a golden brown color.
Add the sausage mixture back, and warm through.
Transfer to serving platter and top with Grana Padano cheese.

Per serving: Cal 834; Fat 62g; Net Carbs 9.5g; Protein 56g

DESSERTS

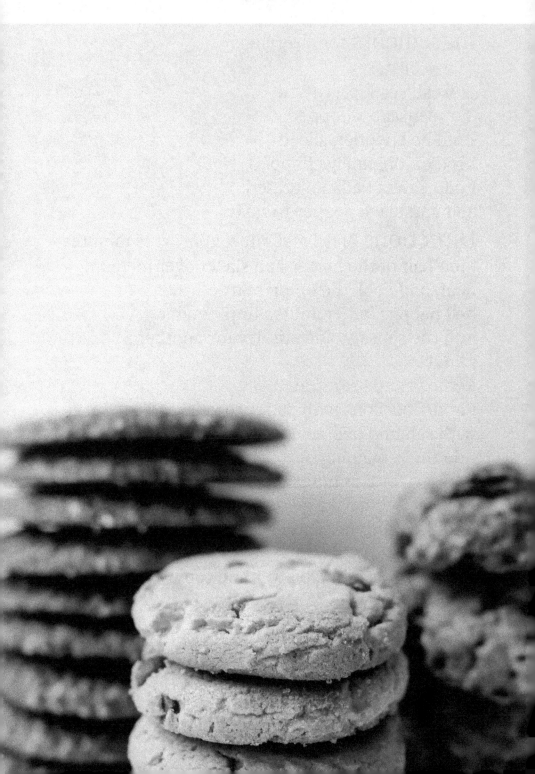

Fluffy Lemon Curd Mousse with Walnuts

Ingredients for 4 servings
For the mousse
1 cup cold heavy cream
8 oz cream cheese
¼ cup swerve sugar
1 tsp vanilla extract
½ lemon, juiced
For the caramel nuts
1 cup walnuts, chopped
2/3 cup swerve brown sugar
A pinch salt
Directions and Total Time: approx. 10 min + chilling time
In a stand mixer, beat cream cheese and heavy cream until creamy.
Add vanilla, swerve sugar, and lemon juice until smooth.
Divide the mixture between 4 dessert cups.
Cover with plastic wrap, and refrigerate for at least 2 hours.

For the caramel walnuts:

Add swerve sugar to a large skillet and cook over medium heat with frequent stirring until melted and golden brown.

Mix in 2 tbsp of water and salt and cook further until syrupy and slightly thickened.

Turn the heat off and quickly mix in the walnuts until well coated in the caramel; let sit for 5 minutes.

Remove the mousse from the fridge and top with the caramel walnuts.

Serve immediately.

Per serving: Cal 521; Net Carbs 8g; Fat 53g; Protein 7g

Chocolate Mousse with Cherries

Ingredients for 4 servings
12 oz unsweetened dark chocolate
8 eggs, separated into yolks and whites
2 tbsp salt
¾ cup swerve sugar
½ cup olive oil
3 tbsp brewed coffee
Cherries
1 cup cherries, pitted and halved
½ stick cinnamon
½ cup swerve sugar
½ cup water
½ lime, juiced
Directions and Total Time: approx. 45 minutes
In a bowl, add the chocolate and melt in the microwave for 95 seconds.
In a separate bowl, whisk the yolks with half of the swerve sugar until a

pale yellow has formed, then, beat in the salt, olive oil, and coffee.

Mix in the melted chocolate until smooth.

In a third bowl, whisk the whites with the hand mixer until a soft peak has formed.

Sprinkle the remaining swerve sugar over and gently fold in with a spatula.

Fetch a tablespoon of the chocolate mixture and fold in to combine.

Pour in the remaining chocolate mixture and whisk to mix.

Ladle the mousse into ramekins, cover with plastic wrap, and refrigerate overnight.

The next day, pour ½ cup of water, ½ cup of swerve, ½ stick cinnamon, and lime juice in a saucepan and bring to a simmer for 4 minutes, stirring to ensure the swerve has dissolved and a syrup has formed.

Add cherries and poach in the sweetened water for 20 minutes until soft.

Turn heat off and discard the cinnamon stick.

Spoon a plum each with syrup on the chocolate mousse and serve.

Per serving: Cal 288; Fat 24g; Net Carbs 8.1g; Protein 10g

Ingredients for 4 servings
1/3 cup ghee
10 saffron threads
1 1/3 cups coconut milk
1 ¾ cups shredded coconut
4 tbsp xylitol
1 tsp cardamom powder
Directions and Total Time: approx. 3 hours
In a bowl, combine the shredded coconut with a cup of coconut milk.
In another bowl, mix together the remaining coconut milk with xylitol and
saffron.
Let sit for 30 minutes.
In a wok, heat the ghee.
Add the coconut mixtures and cook for 5 minutes on low heat, mixing continuously.

Stir in the cardamom and cook for
another 5 minutes.
Spread the mixture onto a small
container and freeze for 2 hours.
Cut into bars to enjoy.
Per serving: Cal 224; Fat 22g; Net
Carbs 2.7g; Protein 3.3g

Chocolate Almond Ice Cream Treats

Ingredients for 4 servings
Ice cream
½ cup heavy whipping cream
½ tsp vanilla extract
½ tsp xanthan gum
¼ cup almond butter
½ cup half and half
1 cup almond milk
¼ tsp stevia powder
½ tbsp vegetable glycerin
2 tbsp erythritol
Chocolate
¾ cup coconut oil
¼ cup cocoa butter pieces, chopped
2 oz unsweetened chocolate
3 ½ tsp THM super sweet blend
Directions and Total Time: approx. 20 min + cooling time
In a bowl, blend all ice cream ingredients until smooth.

Place in an ice cream maker and follow the instructions.

Spread the ice cream into a lined pan, and freezer for about 4 hours.

Mix all chocolate ingredients in a microwave-safe bowl and heat until melted.

Allow cooling.

Remove ice cream from the freezer and slice into bars.

Dip into the cooled chocolate mixture and return to the freezer for about 10 minutes before serving.

Per serving: Cal 305; Fat 25g; Net Carbs 5.3g; Protein 6.2g

Creamy Berry Bowl with Pecans

Ingredients for 4 servings
4 cups Greek yogurt
Liquid stevia to taste
1 ½ cups mascarpone cheese
1 ½ cups blackberries and raspberries
1 cup toasted pecans
Directions and Total Time: approx. 8 minutes
In a bowl, mix the yogurt, stevia, and mascarpone until thoroughly combined.
Divide the mixture into bowls, share the berries and pecans on top of the cream.
Serve immediately.
Per serving: Cal 398; Fat 37.3g; Net Carbs 4.2g; Protein 16g

Hot Chocolate with Almonds & Cinnamon

Ingredients for 4 servings
3 cups almond milk
4 tbsp unsweetened cocoa powder
2 tbsp xylitol
3 tbsp almond butter
Finely chopped almonds to garnish
Ground cinnamon to garnish
Directions and Total Time: approx. 10 minutes
Add the almond milk, cocoa powder, and xylitol in a saucepan, and stir until the sweetener dissolves.
Set the pan over low to heat through for 6 minutes, without boiling.
Swirl the mix occasionally.
Stir in the almond butter until incorporated and turn the heat off.
Transfer the hot chocolate to mugs and sprinkle with almonds and cinnamon, before serving it hot.

Per serving: Cal 273; Fat 20.8g; Net Carbs 8.3g; Protein 10g

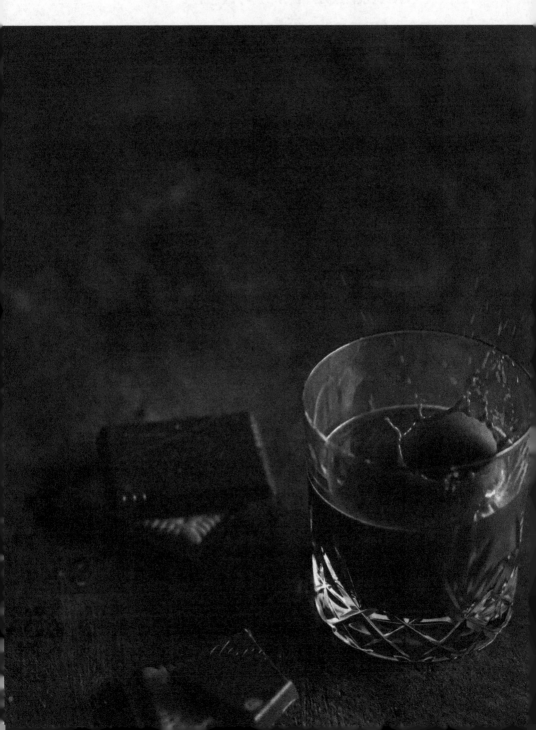

Winter Hot Chocolate with Peanuts

Ingredients for 4 servings
3 tbsp peanut butter
3 cups almond milk
4 tbsp cocoa powder
2 tbsp swerve
Chopped peanuts to garnish
Directions and Total Time: approx. 10 minutes
In a saucepan, add the almond milk, cocoa powder, and swerve.
Stir the mixture until the swerve dissolves.
Set the pan over low to heat through for 5 minutes, without boiling.
Swirl the mix occasionally.
Turn the heat off and stir in the peanut butter until incorporated.
Pour the hot chocolate into mugs and sprinkle with chopped peanuts.
Per serving: Cal 219; Net Carbs 0.8g; Fat 22g; Protein5g

Ingredients for 4 servings
Piecrust
¼ cup almond flour + extra for dusting
3 tbsp coconut flour
½ tsp salt
¼ cup butter, cold and crumbled
3 tbsp erythritol
1 ½ tsp vanilla extract
4 whole eggs
Filling
4 tbsp melted butter
3 tsp swerve brown sugar
1 cup fresh blackberries
1 tsp vanilla extract
1 lemon, juiced
1 cup ricotta cheese
3 to 4 fresh mint leaves to garnish
1 egg, lightly beaten
Directions and Total Time: approx. 50
min + chilling time

In a large bowl, mix the almond flour, coconut flour, and salt.

Add the butter and mix with an electric hand mixer until crumbly.

Add the erythritol and vanilla extract until mixed in.

Then, pour in the 4 eggs one after another while mixing until formed into a ball.

Flatten the dough a clean flat surface, cover in plastic wrap, and refrigerate for 1 hour.

Preheat the oven to 350 F and grease a pie pan with cooking spray.

Lightly dust a clean flat surface with almond flour, unwrap the dough, and roll out the dough into a 1-inch diameter circle.

In a 10-inch shallow baking pan, mix the butter, swerve brown sugar, blackberries, vanilla extract, and lemon juice.

Arrange the blackberries uniformly
across the pan.
Lay the pastry over the fruit filling and
tuck the sides into the pan.
Brush with the beaten egg and bake in
the oven for 35 to 40 minutes or
until the golden and puffed up.
Remove, allow cooling for 5 minutes,
and then run a knife around the pan
to losing the pastry.
Turn the pie over onto a plate,
crumble the ricotta cheese on top,
and
garnish with the mint leaves.
Per serving: Cal 533; Fat 44g; Net
Carbs 8.7g; Protein 17g

Maple-Vanilla Tart

Ingredients for 4 servings
Piecrust
¼ cup almond flour + extra for dusting
3 tbsp coconut flour
½ tsp salt
¼ cup butter, cold and crumbled
3 tbsp erythritol
1 ½ tsp vanilla extract
4 whole eggs
Filling
2 whole eggs + 3 egg yolks
½ cup swerve sugar
1 tsp vanilla bean paste
2 tbsp coconut flour
1 ¼ cup almond milk
1 ¼ cup heavy cream
2 tbsp maple syrup, sugar-free
¼ cup chopped almonds
Directions and Total Time: approx. 75
minutes

Preheat the oven to 350 F and grease a pie pan with cooking spray.
In a large bowl, mix the almond flour, coconut flour, and salt.
Add the butter and mix with an electric hand mixer until crumbly.
Add the erythritol and vanilla extract until mixed in.
Then, pour in the 4 eggs one after another while mixing until formed into a
ball.
Flatten the dough a clean flat surface, cover in plastic wrap, and refrigerate for 1 hour.
After, lightly dust a clean flat surface with almond flour, unwrap the dough, and roll out the dough into a large rectangle, ½ - inch thickness and fit into
a pie pan.
Bake in the oven until golden.
Remove after and allow cooling.

In a large mixing bowl, whisk the whole 3 eggs, egg yolks, swerve sugar, vanilla bean paste, and coconut flour.
Put the almond milk, heavy cream, and maple syrup into a medium pot and bring to a boil over medium heat.
Pour the mixture into the egg mixture and whisk while pouring.
Run the batter through a fine strainer into a bowl and skim off any froth.
Take out the pie pastry from the oven, pour out the baking beans, remove the parchment paper, and transfer the egg batter into the pie.
Bake in the oven for 40 to 50 minutes or until the custard sets with a slight wobble in the center.
Garnish with the chopped almonds, slice, and serve when cooled.
Per serving: Cal 542; Fat 41g; Net Carbs 8.5g; Protein 16g

Ingredients for 4 servings
1 large low carb pie crust
1 ½ cups heavy cream
2 tbsp erythritol + some for topping
1 tbsp culinary lavender
1 vanilla, seeds extracted
2 cups fresh raspberries
Directions and Total Time: approx. 2 hours 25 minutes
Place the pie crust with its pan on a baking tray and bake in a preheated to 380 F oven for 30 minutes, until golden brown; remove and let cool.
In a saucepan over medium heat, mix the heavy cream and lavender, and bring to a boil; turn the heat off and let cool.
Refrigerate for 1 hour to infuse the cream.
Remove the cream from the fridge and strain through a colander into a

bowl to remove the lavender pieces. Mix erythritol and vanilla into the cream, and pour into the cooled crust. Scatter the raspberries on and refrigerate the pie for 45 minutes. Remove and top with erythritol, before slicing.

Per serving: Cal 323; Fat 33.6g; Net Carbs 11.3g; Protein 5.2g

Cinnamon Pumpkin Pie

Ingredients for 4 servings
Crust
6 tbsp butter
2 cups almond flour
1 tsp cinnamon
1/3 cup sweetener
Filling
2 cups shredded pumpkin
¼ cup butter
¼ cup erythritol
½ tsp cinnamon
½ tsp lemon juice
Topping
¼ tsp cinnamon
2 tbsp erythritol
Directions and Total Time: approx. 65 minutes
Combine all crust ingredients in a bowl.
Press this mixture into the bottom of a greased pan.

Bake for 5 minutes in a preheated to 370 F oven.

Meanwhile, in a bowl, combine the pumpkin and lemon juice and let them sit until the crust is ready.

Arrange on top of the crust.

Combine the rest of the filling ingredients, and brush this mixture over the

pumpkin.

Bake for about 35 minutes.

Press the pumpkin down with a spatula, return to oven and bake for 20

more minutes.

Combine the cinnamon and 2 tbsp erythritol, in a bowl, and sprinkle over the tart.

Per serving: Cal 388; Fat 33.6g; Net Carbs 7.6g; Protein 8.5g

Ingredients for 4 servings
Piecrust
¼ cup almond flour + extra for dusting
3 tbsp coconut flour
½ tsp salt
¼ cup butter, cold and crumbled
3 tbsp erythritol
1 ½ tsp vanilla extract
4 whole eggs
Filling
2 ¼ cup strawberries and blackberries
1 cup erythritol + extra for sprinkling
1 vanilla pod, bean paste extracted
1 egg, beaten
Directions and Total Time: approx. 30 min + chilling time
In a large bowl, mix the almond flour, coconut flour, and salt.
Add the butter and mix with an electric hand mixer until crumbly.

Add the erythritol and vanilla extract until mixed in.

Then, pour in the 4 eggs one after another while mixing until formed into a
ball.

Flatten the dough a clean flat surface, cover in plastic wrap, and refrigerate for 1 hour.

Preheat oven to 350 F and grease a pie pan with cooking spray.

Lightly dust a clean flat surface with almond flour, unwrap the dough, and roll out the dough into a large rectangle, ½ - inch thickness and fit into a pie
pan.

Pour some baking beans onto the pastry and bake in the oven until golden.

Remove after, pour pout the baking beans, and allow cooling.

In a bowl, mix the berries, erythritol, and vanilla bean paste.

Spoon the mixture into the pie, level with a spoon, and use the pastry strips to create a lattice top over the berries. Brush with the beaten egg, sprinkle with more erythritol, and bake for 30 minutes or until the fruit is bubbling and the pie golden brown.

Remove from the oven, allow cooling, slice, and serve with whipped cream.

Per serving: Cal 313; Fat 23.5g; Net Carbs 7.3g; Protein 10g

Ingredients for 4 servings
1 cup crushed almond biscuits
½ cup butter, melted
Filling
1 ½ cups mascarpone cheese
¾ cup swerve sugar
1 ½ cups whipping cream
1 tsp vanilla bean paste
4-6 tbsp cold water
1 tbsp gelatin powder
Passionfruit fruit
1 cup passion fruit pulp
¼ cup swerve confectioner's sugar
1 tsp gelatin powder
¼ cup water, room temperature
Directions and Total Time: approx. 2 hours 30 minutes
In a bowl, mix crushed biscuits and butter.
Spoon into a spring-form pan, and use the back of the spoon to level at the

bottom; set aside in the fridge.

In another bowl, put the mascarpone cheese, swerve sugar, and vanilla paste, and whisk with a hand mixer until smooth; set aside.

In a third bowl, add 2 tbsp of cold water and sprinkle 1 tbsp of gelatin powder.

Let dissolve for 5 minutes.

Pour the gelatin liquid and the whipping cream in the cheese mixture and

fold gently.

Remove the spring-form pan from the refrigerator and pour over the mixture.

Return to the fridge.Then, repeat the dissolving process for the remaining gelatin and once your out of ingredients, pour the confectioner's sugar, and

¼ cup of water into it.

Mix and stir in the passion fruit pulp.

Remove the cake again and pour the jelly over it.

Swirl the pan to make the jelly level up.

Place the pan back into the fridge to cool for 2 hours.

When completely set, remove and unlock the spring-pan.

Lift the pan from the cake and slice the dessert.

Per serving: Cal 383; Fat 26g; Net Carbs 6.8g; Protein 9.3g

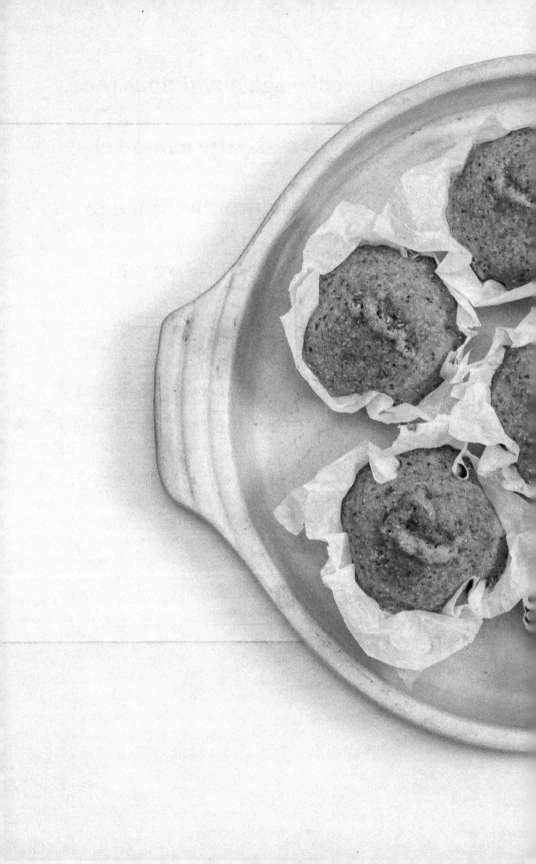

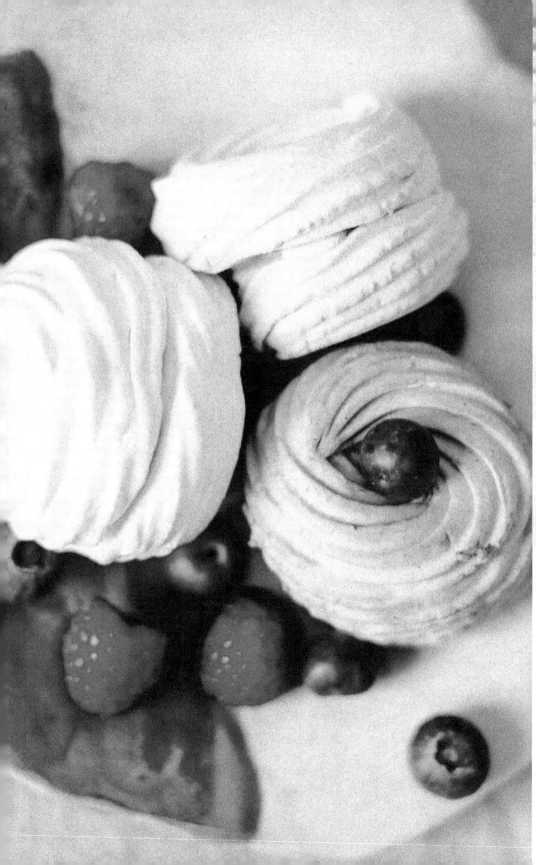

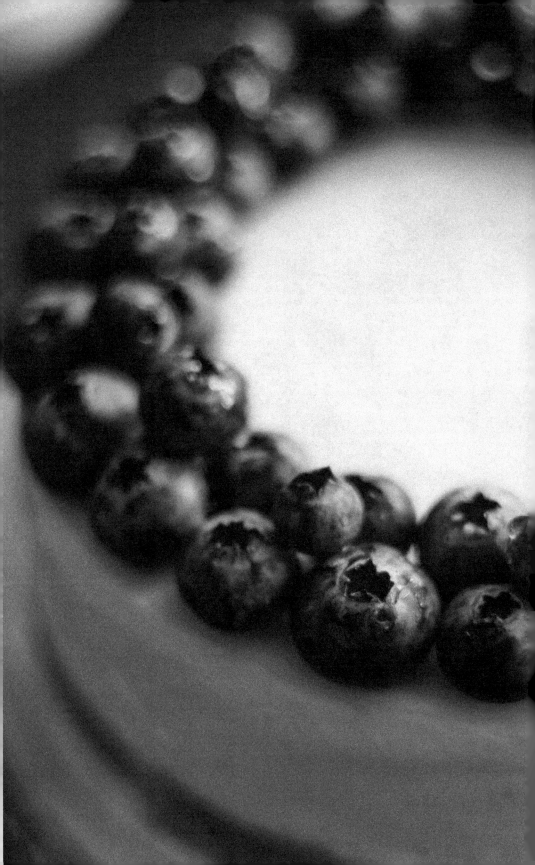

CPSIA information can be obtained
at www.ICGtesting.com
Printed in the USA
BVHW091734150521
607359BV00003B/570

9 781802 533774